High Fiber Foods

How To Lose Weight When On A High Fiber Diet

By: Erik Smith

I0412362

Free Bonus!

Do you want to master your fitness and health so you can feel and look amazing in the next 60 days?

I have a free bonus for you that can help dramatically improve your health and fitness that I think you will like. I have put together a 5-Day email course that will help you look amazing, but more importantly you will also feel great as well.

If that's something you think you would like, sign up to get the emails starting today.

Sign up here - https://enlightenedmanuals.com/5-health-steps/

Free Books Every Week!

Do you want to get notified when I have free books? Then sign up for my newsletter. I will never spam you. I will only send you valuable stuff that you can use to help you improve your life.

Sign up here - https://enlightenedmanuals.com/free-books/

Disclaimer

This guide is for informational purposes only. The author is not a lawyer or an accountant. Any fitness or diet advice is based upon countless hours of research and hands-on application. You should always seek the advice of a professional before acting on something that has been published or recommended. Results may vary, and the accounts depicted in this book are not considered as the "average". Please understand that there are some links in this guide that if accessed I may benefit financially. No part of this publication shall be reproduced, transmitted, or sold in whole or part in any form without prior consent from the author. By reading this guide you agree that the company or the author is not responsible for any injuries that may happen related to this guide. Consult a doctor before making any significant changes to your lifestyle as a result of this guide.

Introduction – What Is Fiber?

What exactly is fiber and how can it help you? In this book that's what I'm going to attempt to show you. I want to give you the things you need to know and how to apply them in your daily life, so you can feel better but more importantly be healthier.

Fiber is essentially the parts of plants that we eat that can't be digested and absorbed into the body. Now that you have the basic understanding of fiber, let's go a little deeper.

There are a couple of things that you need to know in order to get the most out of this book so you can better apply the information in it. First of all there are two different types of fiber that you need to know. The first is called soluble fiber.

Soluble fiber is the kind of fiber that turns into a gel like substance when it goes through your digestive system. This type of fiber slows down the digestive process. That may sound like a bad thing, but as you will learn, that is actually a good thing. Soluble fiber makes you feel like your full longer. This plays a key role in fat loss, which you will be learning about throughout this guide. Foods that have soluble fiber include oats, bran, and certain fruits.

Insoluble fiber is the type of fiber that goes unchanged during the digestive process. This helps regulate digestion, which you will learn the next section of this guide. Unlike soluble fiber, insoluble fiber can't be dissolved into water, which is the main reason why it helps with digestion. A lot of different kinds of grain have a lot of insoluble fiber in them. Vegetables also have a lot of insoluble fiber as well, especially celery, broccoli, and zucchini.

Benefits Of Eating A High Fiber Diet

Lowers Cholesterol Levels – One thing that eating a high fiber diet will help with is lowering your LDL cholesterol level. (Bad cholesterol) The soluble fiber that you find in plants has the ability to help lower your LDL cholesterol. It does this by slowing down the digestive process of fatty acids and helping regulate the release of blood sugars better so that they aren't quickly released. A great article explaining the process better can be found here - http://healthyeating.sfgate.com/fiber-reduce-ldl-5545.html

Helps you Maintain and lose weight – Soluble fiber is great for helping you lose fat; it does this a couple of ways. The first way fiber is good for helping you lose weight is that fiber helps keep the bacteria in your intestine healthy. These bacteria known as Gut Microbiota or just simply Gut Flora has been shown to help regulate your weight and also your blood sugar levels. This is because these bacteria eat the undigested fiber that passes through your digestive system. So essentially if the bacteria in your gut is happy, then you will be happy as well.

Another way fiber helps you lose weight is it helps you decrease your cravings for food. This is because fiber slows down the digestive process of foods tremendously. Because this process takes longer, your body won't tell you it needs food because it is still digesting the food you already ate. Although it has been shown that there are only certain types of fiber that help you with this. Make sure you are eating foods that have fiber that are thicker. Beans for example are thinker than a lot of other types of foods that have fiber in them. A good article to learn more about how fiber can help you lose weight can be found here - http://authoritynutrition.com/fiber-can-help-you-lose-weight/

Digestive Health – The two types of fiber (Soluble and insoluble) play a major part in the digestive process in your body and if you eat the right amount of fiber you will notice a big difference in how you feel. The way that insoluble fiber helps with the digestive process is that it helps the food you eat travel more efficiently and smoothly in the intestines. This means you are less likely to experience constipation and other related conditions. The way that soluble fiber helps with digestion is that it helps your body absorb more nutrients because it slow down the digestive process. So in a sense, you are slowing down the process in order to obtain the blood sugars your body needs, but also fiber helps things run more smoothly.

Skin Health – Fiber does an excellent job in getting rid of toxins in your body. A direct result of this will be great looking skin. Your skin will appear clear and any rashes will go away with a high fiber diet. There are other benefits of flushing out toxins in your body, but the most notable will be in your skin.

High Fiber Foods

Bran – There are actually a lot of types of bran. There's oat bran, corn bran, rice bran, etc. The type of bran that I personally like is corn bran; it has 22g of fiber in 1 ounce. Oat bran and wheat bran only have 12g of fiber in an ounce. Corn bran is also high in insoluble fiber. An easy way to get some bran in your daily diet is to put it on your meals such as your cereal or put it into baked foods such as muffins. Bran muffins are my favorite. There are also many protein bars that already have bran in them as well.

Broccoli – A good vegetable to always have on hand is broccoli. With about 5 grams of fiber per cup, broccoli should be your go to vegetable if you want to increase your fiber intake. Normally I'll just eat broccoli raw, but as you probably know there are so many possible ways to get it into your diet daily. Chicken, broccoli, and ziti is one of my favorite dishes and it's one of my go to plates on the menu at a restaurant. And don't believe someone if they tell you that when you steam or cook broccoli, it loses it's fiber content, it doesn't.

Cabbage – Another green fiber that has a good amount of fiber in it is cabbage. A lot of people don't like cabbage, but I would argue that it's not cabbage itself, but more about how the cabbage is prepared. Only one leaf of cabbage offers over a half of gram of fiber. So just image a whole meal of cabbage! One of the easiest ways to get cabbage in your diet is by ordering coleslaw at restaurants instead of French fries. Or you can simply make coleslaw at home, it's really easy. You could also put it into soup or make corn beef and cabbage.

Raspberries – With 8g of fiber per cup and .08 of fat, raspberries is a great choice if you want to get fiber into your diet and burn some fat. They also have a high amount of vitamin C, manganese, and copper. If you are looking for a good super food that will give you a lot of antioxidant and anti-inflammatory benefits, then raspberries should be at the top of your list. You can eat them by themselves or include them in a fruit salad, which can be a good midmorning snack instead of drinking another cup of coffee.

Romaine Lettuce – I know it's kind of boring, but if you eat enough of this stuff you can increase your fiber content immensely. The easiest way to get romaine lettuce in your diet is to eat a salad or a chicken caesar salad wrap, which are my favorite.

Celery – Here's another simple food that you can eat to get some fiber into your diet. In each stick of celery you will get about .6 grams of fiber. And with a fat content of virtually nothing, it's a great way to burn fat, feel full longer, and get a lot of fiber. Celery has a great amount of vitamin K and other important nutrients that your body needs. A very simple way that I personally like eating celery is putting some peanut butter on a stick and eating it that way.

Squash – All types of squash have a good amount of fiber that you could benefits from, but the most beneficial in my opinion is the Hubbard squash. The hubbard squash has one of the highest fiber contents out of all the squash available. When you eat squash you can also expect to get a lot of vitmin A, vitamin C, and Beta-Carotene. I personally just dice squash up into one-inch cubes, boil it, and mash it. I have found that to be the easiest way to prepare it for eating. You shouldn't just expect to eat squash on Thanksgiving either, make it a year round thing.

Beans - Navy Beans, soybeans, kidney beans, black beans, lima beans. Almost any type of bean that you choose to eat will have a good amount of fiber in it. This means you have the opportunity to include beans to every meal that you eat. Whether it's a side dish or whether it's included in the main dish, you can get a lot of beans in your daily diet without even thinking about it. A way I like to get beans in my diet is eating burritos or other Mexican food.

Mushrooms – I think a lot of people forget about mushrooms, but they are high in fiber and add a unique taste to many dishes that you could potently be eating on a daily bases. I personally like raw mushrooms better, but you can get the fiber benefits whether they are cooked or raw. Salads are a great way to eat them or include them in a savory dish like steak or soup.

Oranges – Another good fruit that you can easily add to your diet are oranges. They are also a great way to get vitamin C as well, but you probably already knew that. A small orange has about 2.3 grams of fiber.

Split peas – From eating one cup of split peas you will get 50 grams of fiber, making them a really good choice to eat all the time. The most famous way to get split peas into your diet is from spilt pea soup, but you can just simply boil them if you don't mind eating bland peas. I'm sure there are also all kinds of recipes that you could find on the Internet that could spice up split peas to make them less boring.

Chickpeas – One tablespoon of chickpeas will give you about 2.2 grams of fiber and at least 35 grams in one cup. They are an easy way to add a lot of fiber into your diet. The easiest way to get some chickpeas into your diet is by eating hummus. Who doesn't like hummus as a dip? You can even dip hummus with other high fiber foods to get even more fiber. You can even put it into a sandwich and other creative dishes. Here is a good article to show you other unique ways you can eat hummus - http://www.lifehack.org/articles/lifestyle/25-different-ways-eat-hummus-5-absolutely-authentic.html

Edamame – You may not be familiar with this food, but you should get to know it because it can provide a good amount of fiber. In one cup of edamame you can expect to consume at least 8 grams of fiber. Edamame looks similar to bean pods, but are actually soybeans that haven't matured fully. A lot of Asian dishes have edamame, but you can also get them by making soups, salads, and many other simple dishes you can make at home. They are also good as a side dish, appetizer or as a snack.

Spelt – Spelt is generally considered a type of grain, which is a good grain source other than wheat. It contains about 19 grams of fiber per cup that you consume. You can get a lot of spelt by eating baked goods that use spelt flour. Pretty simple. There are a lot of recipes and different forms of baked goods you can use to eat spelt. It's a funny name, I know, but if you are looking for a good fiber source, spelt is relatively easy to get.

Steel cut oats – Another really simple way to get fiber into your diet is by eating oatmeal or more specifically, foods that contain steel cut oats. Steel cut oats are also good because it offers a good amount of both soluble and insoluble fiber. Another things about steel cut oats is they are easy to consume by eating oatmeal on a daily basis. I like the instant oatmeal that comes in those portable packages because they only take a couple of minutes to make and you can take them anywhere with you.

Millet – If you have ever giving bird feed to birds, then chances are that you have came into contact with this grain. Although the benefits aren't just for birds, they also provide some good fiber into your diet once you start eating it. It has about 17 grams of dietary fiber in one cup. Millet is great for detoxifying the body because of the presence of antioxidants in it. It also helps when you feel bloated or have an upset stomach. You probably have never even heard of millet before reading this, but you should at least try it out and see if you like it.

Buckwheat Groats – These little things are seeds that come from the buckwheat plant and they are packed with a lot of fiber. Another benefit of buckwheat groats is that they are gluten free. The best way to prepare them is to steam them and put them into side dishes like salads or in main dishes as well. Although you should note that when they are not cooked they become are bitter, so it may be better to cook them on the stove if you don't like to eat things with a bitter taste. Buckwheat grouts are really popular in Eastern European countries as well as the Middle East.

Popcorn – I'm sure you know this food really well. If you have ever gone to the movies then chances are you have had a big bag of this stuff and you probably have some in your cabinet at home right now. In one ounce of popcorn you can find at least 3.6 grams of fiber. I especially like popcorn because you can put extra things in it to add flavor and also more things that have fiber as well. I assure you, you can find at least a couple of things in this guide that you could toss into popcorn to add it's fiber content.

Figs – In five dried figs it's estimated you will consume about 5 grams of fiber. That number includes both soluble and insoluble fiber, making them a great addition to your diet to help the digestive system run smoothly. I would personally recommend you buy dried figs just because they are easier to eat and store in your cabinet, but you could also opt for the fresh kind as well. I love taking figs and other assorted dry fruits when I go for a walk in the park or go hiking on a trail. They provide a great "pick me up" when you doing some type of cardio activity.

Blackberries – I love blackberries not only for their taste, but I also like them because they contain 8 grams of fiber in one cup, making them one of the top fruits that you can eat that are high in fiber. That's roughly about thirty percent of your daily recommended fiber intake. They are also good for making you feel fuller faster and will help you maintain that feeling for a while. So blackberries are great for people looking to lose some extra pounds. The easiest way to consume blackberries is just by eating them straight up, but you can even go ahead and make blackberry jam and other things that these berries go well with.

Avocado – In one cup of avocado you can expect to consume about 10 grams of fiber. Avocados are also famous for containing a lot of good fat, namely unsaturated fat. This is another food that you can put into a lot of dishes.

Pears – A fruit that packs a lot of fiber are pears. There's about 6 grams of fiber in an average sized pear. Most of the fiber you will find in a pear is in the skin, so if you eat pears by taking the skin off them first then you are defeating the purpose of eating them if you are trying to add fiber to your diet. The most common way to eat a pear is to just bite into to it.

Dates – Dates are another example of a fruit that have a lot of fiber. In a cup of chopped dates there is about 12 grams of fiber. You will most likely find them in their fried form, but you can also find them not dried and in their original form. You will most likely eat them as a snack, but they can be used in several dishes. These dishes are popular in many Middle Eastern countries and have been eaten for generations. In their fried form, they kind of look like prunes or raisins, but they tend to be a little more sweeter.

Kumquats – Originally from China, kumquats are similar to other citrus fruits, but they are a little different beyond the surface. One thing that separates them from fruits like oranges is they are much smaller. Another thing that many people may not know about kumquats is that you can eat the outside peels. Along with fiber, kumquats are packed with antioxidants and essential oils as well.

Chia Seeds – In an ounce of chia seeds there are about 10 grams of fiber. These seeds, originally from South America are a great way to get your daily fiber into your diet. They are also good for energy boosts as well. Chia seeds are good for people wanting to lose weight because they have the ability to make you feel full faster and for longer time periods. Almost half of the weight in chia seeds is in fiber. They also have a lot of protein and omega 3 fatty acids. To many, chia seeds are considered a "superfood" because of the health properties. There are many other benefits that chia seeds can provide for you, but they are out of the scope of this guide.

Flaxseed – There's about 3 grams of fiber in a tablespoon of flaxseed. You probably have heard of flaxseed in the oil form, but what I'm talking about are the actual seeds in whole form. Although you can still benefit greatly from the oil form of flaxseed, you will get much more fiber content in it's original form. Here is another type of food that has many benefits other than providing fiber. Many people use flaxseed to help with acne, sore throat, constipation, high blood pressure, and many other conditions.

Almonds – In one cup of sliced almonds you get about 11 grams of fiber. Nuts are many people's go to snack, especially almonds. Almonds provide a good energy boost, but also are high in fiber. They are easy to eat if you need fiber and you are in a rush. They also are easy to carry with you and can also be added to homemade trail mix.

Sunflower Seeds – In one cup of sunflower seeds there is 12 grams of fiber. Just like almonds, sunflower seeds are also easy to carry and can be mixed with other high fiber snacks to get even more fiber into your diet. Or just simply grab a handful of them while you're on your way out the door. I also like adding them to cottage cheese to give it more flavor and texture.

Pistachios – In one cup of pistachios there is about 13 grams of fiber. The thing that I like about pistachios, which some people might find a hindrance, is that they come with their shells still attached to them. I like this because it allows be to eat them more slowly, which makes me appreciate the taste of them more and I usually eat less as a result.

Parsnips – In one cup of sliced parsnips there is about 6 grams of fiber and they only have about 100 calories by the same measurement. A parsnip is a root, closely related to carrots and they have many nutrients and vitamins just like carrots do. They are kind of boring by themselves so it is best to find a good recipe that includes several ingredients to make them more exciting, but either way you can get a lot of fiber if you eat them regularly.

Sweet Potato – In a cup of chopped sweet potatoes you will find about 4 grams of fiber. Which isn't that much but chances are you will be eating more than a cup in one sitting, so you will probably be consuming a lot more than just 4 grams at a time. Sweet potatoes are sometimes also called yams. The easiest way to get some sweet potatoes into your diet is to replace them for when you eat regular potatoes. In my opinion they actually taste better anyway.

Whole Wheat Pasta – The biggest difference between whole wheat pasta and regular white pasta is that whole wheat contains more of the grain and more of it is included during the refinement process. This means you will get more fiber when you eat whole grain compared to its regular counterpart.

Spinach – Spinach is one of my all time favorite things to eat and it should be one of your staples in your fridge. This is because spinach has .7 grams of fiber in one cup. That may not seem like much but if you put into account how little carbohydrate you consume when eating spinach, you can basically eat as much as you want. It also has many beneficial nutrients, vitamins, minerals, and many phytonutrients as well. There are many dishes that taste great with spinach and you can eat it anytime of the day without getting weird looks from the people around you. Eat spinach in an omelet or have it as a late night snack if you are into that sort of thing.

Quinoa – With about 12 grams of fiber in one cup, quinoa is a great food to eat when you are trying to add some fiber to your diet. These seeds are packed with a lot of fiber, but they also contain many important nutrients that your body needs such things as magnesium, copper, iron, zinc, and potassium. Quinoa is also gluten free. You'll typically find quinoa in salads, but it can also be used in stuffed peppers and many other dishes as well.

Sesame seeds – In one tablespoon you can expect to find about 1.1 grams of fiber. You probably have had them eating Chinese food or some other type of Asian food. Sesame seed oil is also beneficial not just for it's fiber content but useful for cooking as well. These seeds are high in copper, manganese, calcium, and phosphorus also. Sesame seeds can be sprinkled on almost anything that you seem fit. They have a delicate nutty taste so they usually taste good with anything without ruining the flavor of other foods. They also provide a texture that makes meals more appealing as well.

Pumpkin seeds – Another type of seed that are high in fiber are pumpkin seeds. In a cup of pumpkin seeds there is about 12 grams of fiber. You can roast them and eat them that way or you can include them in various meals. You also can make flour from them as well.

Kale – In recent years kale has gained a lot in popularity. In a cup of chopped kale there is about 2.6 grams of fiber. You can put kale into salads, put them into smoothies, or just eat it raw by itself. If you want to try it in kale, check out my guide on green smoothies here - http://www.amazon.com/gp/product/B00VSCS4VQ

How To Lose Weight From A High Fiber Diet

Before I go into the topic of losing weight from eating fiber, I have to stress one thing and that is just eating fiber alone won't get you to lose weight. You still have to do other things in order to help you burn fat. So if you think you can only eat a lot of fiber and think you will magically start shedding pounds, then your kidding yourself.

There are certain things that you need to make sure you do in order to burn those calories, plus have a high fiber diet on top of everything else.

Less calories in, more calories out – The basic concept that you have to understand if you want to lose weight is the input and output of calories. In very basic terms, fat loss happens because you have a deficit of calories. This naturally means that you will burn calories that are stored as fat. So this means you should focus on eating less calories. But doing this without some sort of plan, will lead to an unhealthy lifestyle. There are some diets that I recommend you check out, that are healthy and they also help you to burn fat really efficiently. One diet that I recommend to anyone who asks me how to lose weight is intermittent fasting. When on this diet, (which really isn't a diet at all) you have a window an eating period and then you fast for the remaining of the day. Much of the details about this diet are out of the scope of this guide, but if you want to learn more about intermittent fasting, check out my other guide here - http://www.amazon.com/gp/product/B00U39VVHY

Don't drink calories – A common mistake as lot of people as when tried to lose weight is they drink sugary drinks and drinks that have a lot of calories. When you drink things that have a lot of calories, it is more likely that your body will store those calories as fat, rather than those calories burning burned as energy. Your body doesn't really need to break down those liquid calories as much, so it makes it easy on the body, which isn't what you want if you want to burn fat. So I suggest the majority of the things you drink to be only water. Sure, you can have black coffee and other drinks that don't have that many calories or sugar in them, but you should avoid most drinks because they won't help you lose weight.

Exercise – The last thing I recommend you do if you want to lose weight and to help aid your high fiber diet is to exercise effectively. What I mean by efficiently is you don't need to go overboard with your workouts. If you simply workout two to three times a week, that is perfect. You don't need to spend countless hours at the gym and you certainly don't need to workout everyday. Two things you should focus on while at the gym are cardio and building muscle. Cardio as you probably know burn a great deal of calories, but it can get pretty boring. In order to combat that, here are a few things you can do to change up your boring cardio routine; biking, jumping rope, swimming, kick boxing, or simply walking around your neighborhood.

The second thing that you should focus on is building muscle. This is because the more muscle you have the more calories your body will burn to help maintain that muscle. It takes a lot of energy to maintain muscle, so you should expect to see more calories being burned, the more muscle you have on your body. To do this you should weight lift, using heavy weight. The majority of your weight lifting routine should be using compound exercises. These are exercises that use more than one muscle group. Exercises like squats, deadlift, and bench press are all examples of compound exercises. These will give you the best results without spending too much time in the gym.

Things you can do to add fiber to your diet

Eat oatmeal or cereal for breakfast – A great way to start the day is to eat a bowl of oatmeal or a healthy cereal that is high in fiber. This does a couple of things that are beneficial to you, especially if you are looking to lose weight. The first thing this does is it will help you to feel full throughout the morning. You will feel a lot more full if you eat a bowl of cereal or oatmeal, rather than eating some of type of food, or even worse; when you don't eat anything for breakfast at all. You will be able to go longer in the day without having to eat a snack or your lunch because you won't feel hungry as much, aiding your ability to take in less calories which promotes weight loss. Another thing eating a high fiber breakfast will help you is help promote healthy digestive function through your day. After you have fasted while you were sleeping during the night, you weren't eating anything, which may lead to bloating. But if you eat fiber first thing in the morning you can avoid all that and kick start the digestive process.

Add it to every meal – Every meal you have, you should make sure you include a food that id high in fiber. I gave you a list of the foods that have the highest amount of fiber that you can find in this guide, so pick just a few and include them into your daily diet. Even if you go out to restaurants, make sure you are eating high fiber foods.

Snack on high fiber foods rather than sweets – Another simple tip, one that is pretty straight forward is when you feel like a snack make sure you are eating foods that have a lot of fiber in them. This may seem obvious to a lot of people reading this, but there are so many people out there that don't do this and it shows by their ability to lose weight. A great article that I recommend you check out with some really cool snack ideas that have a lot of fiber in them can be found here - http://greatist.com/health/high-fiber-snacks

Salads – The foods that you find in salads usually are high in fiber. Lettuce among the other common things you find in salads make it a meal that you should consume regularly. You can find a lot of salad recipes online that have many ingredients that are high in fiber. Or you can create your own salads by adding foods that you find in this guide that you would like to try.

Soups - Eating soup is also another great option to help add some fiber into your diet.

Conclusion

So there you have it, some useful tips that you can use starting today that will get you closer to your goal of losing weight using the power of fiber. I hope in this quick guide you have learned some things that can help you achieve your fitness and health goals much faster. The journey may not always be that easy, but if you have a plan and execute it everyday, then the process will be simple to follow.

Free Bonus!

Do you want to master your fitness and health so you can feel and look amazing in the next 60 days?

I have a free bonus for you that can help dramatically improve your health in fitness that I think you will like. I have put together a 5-Day email course that will help you look amazing, but more importantly you will also feel great as well.

If that's something you think you would like, sign up to get the emails starting today.

Sign up here - https://enlightenedmanuals.com/5-health-steps/

Free Books Every Week!

Do you want to get notified when I have free books? Then sign up for my newsletter. I will never spam you. I will only send you valuable stuff that you can use to help you improve your life.

Sign up here - https://enlightenedmanuals.com/free-books/